# HERBS FOR HIGH CHOLESTEROL

## An essential guide on herds to treat high cholesterol

**Dr Rowan Theo**

**Table of Contents**

# CHAPTER ONE

## Natural Remedies for High Cholesterol

Natural or complementary remedies for coronary heart disorder frequently purpose to manipulate levels of cholesterol, decrease blood stress, and enhance coronary heart fitness. Typically, studies on such remedies is limited, as compared with that of traditional clinical remedies.

Few herbal merchandise have had sufficient studies performed to show they are able to lessen ldl cholesterol clinically.

However, many human beings have skilled a few achievement with opportunity remedies, and a few ldl cholesterol-reducing dietary supplements and herbal treatments is probably useful.

Before you attempt any opportunity remedies, take a look at with a healthcare expert to decide if they're secure for you. The components in a few opportunity treatment options can intrude with sure medicinal drugs or have dangerous facet consequences.

## 1. Astragalus

Astragalus is an herb used to guide the immune gadget in conventional Chinese medication. It has antibacterial and anti inflammatory properties. It's taken into consideration to be an "adaptogen." This manner it's believed to shield the frame in opposition to numerous stresses.

Limited research advise that astragalus may also have a few blessings to your coronary heart. But in keeping with the National Center for Complementary and Integrative Health (NCCIH), excessive first-rate scientific human trials are usually lacking. More studies is wanted to learn the way astragalus may also have an effect on your levels of cholesterol and average coronary heart fitness.

## 2. Hawthorn

Hawthorn is a shrub associated with the rose. Its berries, leaves, and flora had been used for coronary heart troubles for the reason that Roman Empire.

Some research have observed the plant to be an powerful remedy for milder kinds of coronary heart failure. However, studies outcomes are conflicting, warns the NCCIH. There's now no longer sufficient clinical proof to recognize if hawthorn is powerful for different coronary heart troubles.

Also, hawthorn could have terrible interactions with many prescription medicinal drugs and different herbs.

## 3 Flax seed

Flax seed comes from the flax plant. Both flax seed and flaxseed oil include excessive ranges of alpha-linolenic acid (ALA). This is an omega-three fatty acid that could assist decrease your chance of coronary heart disorder.

Research at the blessings of flaxseed for coronary heart fitness has produced combined results, reviews the NCCIH. Some research advise that flaxseed arrangements may also assist decrease ldl cholesterol, specifically amongst human beings with excessive levels of cholesterol and postmenopausal women.

Healthier consuming should not be a hassle. We'll ship you our proof-primarily based totally pointers on meal making plans and nutrition.

## 4. Fish oil dietary supplements with omega-three fatty acids

Omega-three fatty acids also are observed in fish and fish oils. Salmon, tuna, lake trout, herring, sardines, and different fatty fish are particularly wealthy sources.

Experts have lengthy believed that omega-three fatty acids in fish assist lessen the chance of having coronary heart disorder. Other vitamins in fish, or a aggregate of these vitamins and omega-three fatty acids, may also assist shield your coronary heart. Eating one or servings of fatty fish every week may also decrease your possibilities of getting a coronary heart assault.

If you've got coronary heart disorder, you can additionally advantage from taking omega-three fatty acid dietary supplements or consuming different ingredients wealthy in omega-three fatty acids. For example, walnuts, canola oil, and soybeans are top sources. Evidence is more potent for the blessings of consuming fish with omega-three fatty acids than taking dietary supplements or consuming different ingredients.

# CHAPTER TWO

## Red yeast rice

Red yeast rice is a conventional Chinese medication and cooking aspect. It's made with the aid of using culturing pink rice with yeast.

Some pink yeast rice merchandise include vast portions of monacolin K. This substance is chemically equal to the lively aspect in the ldl cholesterol-reducing drug lovastatin. Red yeast rice merchandise that include this substance may also assist lower your blood levels of cholesterol.

Other pink yeast rice merchandise include little to no monacolin K. Some additionally include a contaminant known as citrinin. This contaminant can motive kidney failure.

In many cases, there's no manner that allows you to recognize which merchandise include monacolin K or citrinin. Therefore, it's tough to inform which merchandise may be powerful or secure.

## 6. Plant sterol and stanol dietary supplements

Plant sterols and stanols are materials observed in lots of end result, vegetables, nuts, seeds, grains, and different plants. Some processed ingredients also are fortified with plant sterols or stanols, consisting of fortified margarine, orange juice, or yogurt merchandise.

Plant sterols and stanols may also assist decrease your chance of coronary heart disorder. They assist save you your small gut from soaking up ldl cholesterol. This can decrease LDL (terrible) levels of cholesterol to your blood.

## 7. Garlic

Garlic is an safe to eat bulb that's been used as a cooking aspect and medication for lots of years. It may be eaten uncooked or cooked. It's additionally to be had in complement shape, as a pill or tablet.

Some studies shows that garlic may also assist decrease your blood stress, lessen your blood levels of cholesterol, and gradual the development of atherosclerosis, reviews NCCIH.

However, as with many opportunity treatment options, research have yielded combined results. For example, a few research have observed that taking garlic for 1 to a few months facilitates decrease blood levels of cholesterol.

However, an NCCIH-funded examine at the protection and effectiveness of 3 garlic arrangements observed no lengthy-time period impact on blood ldl cholesterol.

## Pros and cons of herbal treatments

### Pros of herbal treatments

• Most herbal treatments may be accessed with out a prescription.

• Some human beings locate herbal treatments useful while

used with their preferred remedy plan.

Cons of herbal treatments

• There's no proof that opportunity or natural treatments on my own can decrease ldl cholesterol.

• Most herbal treatments are unregulated, because of this that that a few facet consequences can be unknown.

Diet and way of life changes

**You also can undertake wholesome way of life behavior to assist manipulate your blood levels of cholesterol. For example:**

• If you smoke, remember quitting.

• Maintain a wholesome weight to your frame kind.

• Try to exercising maximum days of the week.

• Include greater coronary heart-wholesome ingredients and ingredients wealthy in soluble fiber and omega-three fatty acids.

• Limit your intake of ingredients excessive in saturated fat. For example, replacement olive oil for butter.

• Consider removing trans fat out of your weight loss plan.

• If you drink, make sure it's in moderation.

• Take steps to lessen stress.

## Medications for excessive ldl cholesterol

A form of medicinal drugs also are to be had to decrease excessive ldl cholesterol. For example, your medical doctor may also prescribe:

• statins (lovastatin, atorvastatin)

• ldl cholesterol absorption inhibitors (cholestyramine)

• injectable medicinal drugs (evolocumab)

## The takeaway

Cholesterol is a sort of fats to your blood. Although your frame makes all of the ldl cholesterol it wishes, you furthermore may get ldl cholesterol from the ingredients you eat. Your genetics, age, weight loss plan, pastime ranges, and different elements have an effect on your chance of growing excessive ldl cholesterol.

High ldl cholesterol is one of the foremost chance elements for coronary heart disorder. It will increase your threat of growing coronary heart disorder and having a coronary heart assault. It also can increase your chance of stroke. In particular, excessive ranges of low-density lipoprotein (LDL) ldl cholesterol increase your chance of those situations. LDL ldl cholesterol is frequently known as "terrible" ldl cholesterol.

If you've got excessive ldl cholesterol, your medical doctor may also prescribe medicinal drugs or way of life changes. For example, preserving a wholesome weight to your frame size, growing your bodily pastime, consuming nutrient-wealthy ingredients, and quitting smoking can assist carry your levels of cholesterol down.

# CHAPTER THREE

## Herbs and Supplements to Lower Cholesterol

Many human beings with excessive ldl cholesterol are seeking for numerous approaches to lessen ranges of low-density lipoprotein, LDL or "terrible ldl cholesterol," due to the fact it's far a primary chance aspect for coronary heart disorder and stroke.1Herbs and dietary supplements to decrease ldl cholesterol are a few alternatives they'll remember.

In a few cases, herbs and dietary supplements can be used in conjunction with greater conventional treatment options to attain this goal. So far, though, the clinical guide for the declare that they are able to appropriately be used to deal with excessive ldl cholesterol isn't that firm.

This article explains why ldl cholesterol is this sort of fitness hassle and what is understood approximately how dietary supplements may assist. It additionally seems at who may also advantage from taking dietary supplements, and what merchandise they must select from.

**Good and Bad Cholesterol**

Cholesterol is a sort of waxy fats that your liver makes or which you take in from ingredients. Your frame wishes it due to the fact it's far a key constructing block of your cells. It is likewise had to make hormones and a few digestive fluids.

In a few human beings, though, the levels of cholesterol in the blood turn out to be too excessive. But excessive ldl cholesterol is a time period that wishes teasing out.

Not all excessive levels of cholesterol are problematic. It all relies upon at the composition of your overall ldl cholesterol end result.

Total ldl cholesterol is the sum of varieties of ldl cholesterol, similarly to different lipids:

• Low-density lipoprotein (LDL): Known as "terrible ldl cholesterol," LDL builds up and might motive harm to the liner of blood vessels. This may also make a contribution to atherosclerosis, normally referred to as hardening of the arteries, in addition to different fitness issues.

• High-density lipoprotein (HDL): This kind facilitates circulate different ldl cholesterol from the frame, reducing the chance of terrible fitness consequences it could motive. Because of this, HDL is noted as "top ldl cholesterol."

It's the excessive ranges of low-density lipoprotein (LDL) which can be worrisome. And at the same time as you can have a excessive overall ldl cholesterol due to excessive LDL, it is also feasible to have a ordinary overall ldl cholesterol and excessive LDL.

High ldl cholesterol can be identified if:2

- LDL ldl cholesterol is over one hundred milligrams in step with deciliter (mg/dL)

- HDL ldl cholesterol is beneath 60 mg/dL

- Total ldl cholesterol is over two hundred mg/dL

What's taken into consideration a wholesome or regarding end result for you can fluctuate from this primarily based totally on elements like your age and own circle of relatives fitness records.

Low LDL and excessive HDL numbers are typically the goal dreams for remedy and way of life changes.

## Who Can Take Supplements

Researchers are nevertheless in search of to verify the blessings of dietary supplements in treating excessive ldl cholesterol. For this motive, it stays doubtful who can or can not take them. In general, they may be taken into consideration more secure to apply in more youthful human beings without a records of great coronary heart-associated contamination or chance.

However, anyone ought to talk to a healthcare issuer earlier than taking dietary supplements.

One motive for that is due to the fact your very own clinical records may also encompass different fitness situations that can be stricken by taking an herb or dietary complement.

Another situation can be the ability for interplay with any pills you already take.

# CHAPTER FOUR

## Recap

Supplements can be one choice for improving "top" HDL levels of cholesterol, reducing "terrible" LDL ranges, and, in turn, decreasing the chance of stroke and coronary heart-associated contamination. While studies has proven that a few merchandise may also assist to decrease ldl cholesterol, their blessings aren't but proven. It's essential to talk on your healthcare issuer earlier than beginning one.

## Niacin (Vitamin B3)

Niacin, a shape of diet B3 additionally known as nicotinic acid, is used to decrease ldl cholesterol. It seems that niacin lowers LDL ldl cholesterol and triglycerides, and raises "top" HDL ldl cholesterol. Niacin additionally seems to seriously decrease ranges for some other chance aspect of atherosclerosis, known as lipoprotein A.

Niacin can boom the impact of excessive blood stress medication. It additionally may also motive nausea, indigestion, gas, diarrhea, or gout. It can get worse peptic ulcers, and cause liver infection or excessive blood sugar.

The maximum common facet impact of excessive-dose niacin is pores and skin flushing or warm flashes. This is as a result of the widening of blood vessels. Most human beings handiest observe this after they first of all begin taking niacin. The flushing signs may also ease if niacin is thinking about food.

Some researchers have proposed that excessive doses of niacin may assist to decrease ldl cholesterol while blended with normally used pills known as statins. However, different research have proven no scientific advantage from doing so, or even recommended the opportunity of a few harm. The technology is inconclusive, so that they should not be blended except beneath the near supervision of a healthcare issuer.

Because of facet consequences, niacin ought to now no longer be used to decrease ldl cholesterol except beneath the supervision of a certified fitness practitioner.

## Soluble Fiber

Soluble fiber seems to decrease ldl cholesterol with the aid of using decreasing the quantity of ldl cholesterol this is absorbed in the intestines.

Soluble fiber is the type that binds with ldl cholesterol in order that it's far excreted from the frame. It may be observed as a nutritional complement, consisting of psyllium powder, or in ingredients consisting of:

• Oats, barley, rye

• Legumes (peas, beans)

• Some end result consisting of apples, prunes, and berries

• Some vegetables, consisting of carrots, broccoli, and yams

• Carob

Five to ten grams an afternoon of soluble fiber has been observed to decrease LDL ldl cholesterol with the aid of using about five%.

Other dietary supplements and ingredients excessive in soluble fiber encompass acacia fiber, shirataki noodles, nopal, and flaxseeds.

## Plant Sterols and Stanols

Plant stanols and sterols, consisting of beta-sitosterol, are naturally-happening materials observed in sure plants. Stanols also are observed as nutritional dietary supplements. Some are delivered to margarine, orange juice, and dressings.

Research shows that plant stanols and sterols may also assist to decrease ldl cholesterol. They are comparable in chemical shape and might assist block the absorption of ldl cholesterol in the intestines. The National Cholesterol Education Program recommends you are taking in 2 grams of plant sterols and stanols every day.6

lets in an permitted fitness declare on phytosterols stating, "Foods containing as a minimum 0.sixty five gram in step with serving of vegetable oil plant sterol esters, eaten two times an afternoon with food for a every day overall consumption of as a minimum 1.three grams, as a part of a weight loss plan low in saturated fats and ldl cholesterol, may also lessen the chance of coronary heart disorder."

Stanols and sterols seem to decorate the consequences of different techniques to decrease ldl cholesterol. In research, human beings taking statin pills to decrease ldl cholesterol had an extra development of their levels of cholesterol with stanols/sterols.

## Artichoke Leaf

There is a few studies suggesting that artichoke leaf extract (Cynara scolymnus) may also assist to decrease ldl cholesterol.7 Artichoke leaf extract may match with the aid of using restricting the synthesis of ldl cholesterol in the frame.

Artichokes additionally include a compound known as cynarine. It is thought to boom bile manufacturing in the liver and velocity the go with the drift of bile from the gallbladder. Both of those movements may also increase ldl cholesterol excretion.

However, research have proven the proof for the use of artichoke leaf isn't but convincing and greater studies is wanted.

# CHAPTER FIVE

## Other Supplements

Other dietary supplements which have been recommended for ldl cholesterol have much less proof of being useful.

Garlic has now been proven to be useless for reducing ldl cholesterol. Other dietary supplements and meals you can see touted encompass policosanol, which may also provide blessings for controlling levels of cholesterol, however the studies outcomes continue to be inconclusive.

More studies additionally is wanted to look if coenzyme Q10 facilitates to restrict hardening of the arteries, frequently connected to ldl cholesterol buildup and associated coronary heart-fitness issues.

Studies additionally advise that catechin compounds in inexperienced tea may also assist to lessen the frame's absorption of ldl cholesterol. Soy, too, has been observed to expose blessings in reducing ldl cholesterol, however maximum research have observed minimum consequences.

In the case of pink yeast rice, there's a ability threat as it includes a naturally-happening shape of lovastatin, a prescription drug.

## Modifying Risk Behaviors

High ldl cholesterol is typically dealt with primarily based totally on overall ldl cholesterol, LDL ldl cholesterol, and HDL levels of cholesterol, plus the presence of extra chance elements for coronary heart disorder.

While a few chance elements can not be changed, others can. These chance elements may also encompass:

• Previous coronary heart assault

• Diabetes

• Smoking

• High blood stress

• Low HDL ldl cholesterol

• Family records of early coronary heart disorder

• Age over forty five in guys and extra than fifty five in women

• 10-yr chance of a coronary heart assault extra than 20%

Of those, now no longer smoking (or quitting in case you smoke) is some thing you may take motion on. You also can deal with your excessive blood stress and diabetes to preserve them beneath control.

## Using Alternative Medicine

Before making a decision to apply opportunity medication for excessive ldl cholesterol, observe those pointers:

• Talk on your healthcare issuer earlier than beginning any herbal approach to decrease ldl cholesterol.

• Make positive your healthcare issuer is aware of what dietary supplements you're taking.

• Don't forestall taking any current pills to decrease ldl cholesterol.

Speak on your healthcare issuer when you have questions on your medication.

• Alternative medication hasn't been examined for protection. Keep this in thoughts while thinking about dietary supplements in pregnant women, nursing mothers, and children. Safety additionally isn't sure for people with clinical situations or who're taking medicinal drugs.

## Summary

People who're worried approximately excessive ldl cholesterol may also remember taking dietary supplements. This may also suggest attempting those merchandise on my own or in aggregate with conventional medication.

Either manner, it is essential to make certain you talk on your healthcare issuer approximately taking niacin, soluble fiber, or one of the different alternatives.

It's additionally essential to recollect that the technology on how secure or powerful those herbal merchandise are nevertheless isn't always settled. More studies is wanted to recognize how dietary supplements may also assist to decrease levels of cholesterol.

# THE END

www.ingramcontent.com/pod-product-compliance
Lightning Source LLC
Chambersburg PA
CBHW071014290526
45795CB00005B/1793